Studies of GENETIC-COMPLEX of Ayurvedic Plants

Indian Medical Science Series No. 46

Studies of GENETIC-COMPLEX of Ayurvedic Plants

Dr. C.R. Karnick
M.D.; Ph.D.; D.Sc.

Sri Satguru Publications
A Division of
Indian Books Centre
Delhi - India

Published by:
Sri Satguru Publications
Indological and Oriental Publishers
A Division of
Indian Books Centre
40/5, Shakti Nagar,
Delhi-110007
(INDIA)

First Edition: Delhi, 1996

ISBN 81-7030-480-6

Printed at . D.K. Fine Art Press (P) Ltd., Delhi-110052

Printed in India.

This work is dedicated
to
My Mother Kamashya Goddess
of Gauhati

Contents

Acknowledgements

I wish to acknowledge, the co-operation and encouragement I have received from a large number of my fellow Scientist colleagues in my Country and Abroad.

My thanks are also due to the Director, Central Council for Research in Ayurveda and Siddha, Govt of India, Ministry of Health and Family Welfare, New Delhi for encouragement.

I record my gratefulness to several of my colleagues of Jawaharlal Nehru Ayurvedic Research Institute and Garden, Pune, the members of Kew Gardens, London, and National Botanical Herbarium, Dehra Dun for confirmation and germplasm studies of plant species.

Also my thanks are due to various Research Institutes and Centres of CCRAS, Jhansi, Gwalior, Guwahati, Bundelkhand University Medical College, Jhansi, Patiala Medical College, Patiala and other medical colleagues of Laboratory, Hospital and O P D for various clinical evaluation of medicinal plants.

Nearly 500 species were studied for their germ-complex. (Chromosomes). Sometimes we observed, polyploids and tetraploid species etc. Plants, were analysed for active principles using latest Chromatographic methods using HPTLC. etc.

Finally I acknowledge my thanks to the Chairman and Managing Director Mr. H.F. Khorakiwala Wockhardt Ltd. for continuous help during the tenure of this research project.

Dr. C.R. Karnick

Research Scientist and Ex. Asst. Director CCRAS

Ministry of Health and Family Welfare,

Govt of India, New Delhi,

Clinical and Exp. Ayurvedic Research Division

Wockhardt, Aurangabad

1

Introduction

India is a subcontinent having large coastal areas, hills and mountain, flat land with several rivers like Indus, Ganges, Tawi, Cauvery and Narmada flowing into its vast area.

Here we have varied temperature complex-Temperate regions in Himalayas with warm tropical areas in flat lands of U.P., M.P., Maharashtra, Karnataka etc. Therefore here we see plants of various types.

The medicinal plants are sources of many biologically active constituents which one cannot ignore by modern Medical practice, due to the fact of having healing effects.

Some of them show unknown features and complexity because of their active constituents which are difficult to prepare synthetically and excessive expensive viz. glycosides gunseng, ergot alkaloids etc.

There are certain plant species like *Solanum*–which contain special constituents that cannot be applied directly for healing but are used as basic materials for semi synthetic processes in pharmacological industry (viz. Corticosteriods).

As opposed to the simple uses of some synthetic materials, the use of drugs is more sophisticated, including the application of essential oils for healing, flavouring, as a part of bio-pharmacology (galeniss teas, biocosmetics).

In certain areas of the chemical industry (viz. Cosmetics, household chemicals), in the food industry, the essential oils extracted from plants cannot be replaced and these are the initial basic materials for producing a new scent or flavour.

The food industry has wide application areas. The advanced diet requires a variety of spices using salt, paprika and pepper, and more people realize the advantageous effects of natural spices on the digestive system.

The study of gene-complex of drug plants is therefore necessary. This will prevent Gene exploitation.

2

Biological Aspects

Plants are living organism and biological phenomena are closely tot he chemical and physical characteristics of macromolecules occurring in living organisms. Their dynamic equilibrium may be attributed to the alterations which continuously occur in the living organisms to the specified enzymes which control these alterations, and to the different natures, ratios and activities of the enzymes, which control these alterations, and to the different natures, ratios and the activities of the enzymes depending on well-defined conditions.

Enzymes are source of inherited characters, because the sun of chemical qualities the *Chemism* which is a system of biochemical processes and is characteristic of the organism. This includes DNA and RNA being the bearers of genetic information and having the ability to transcribe and translate it (cf Protein biosynthesis). Proteins (enzyme stock), as well as the general steps of metabolism (photosynthesis, respiration) and further steps of metabolism (i.e. biosynthesis, accumulation, decomposition of alkaloids, flavonoids, terpenes etc.).

The (intrinsic) reaction of the living in an organism at a certain stage of phylogeny is directly connected with its chemism. The differentiation of any taxon is fundamentally a chemical process. In molecular biology-the so called enzyme stock can be traced back to composition and structure of the proteins of cells, which are the fundamentals of all inherited properties. The basis of the differentiation of cells is found in chemo-differentiation at a molecular level. The fundamental differences appear in course of ontogeny manifest themselves mainly in the differences between proteins present in the organism which is difference between enzyme system.

As per Mothes (1957)-genetics of genetics of metabolism

begins when genetical analysis of collection of races chemically differing from each other.

It is experimentally shown as early as 1950's that it is not possible to produce viable alkaloid-free individuals of any alkaloid bearing species by irradiation.

End products of metabolic processes, if accumulated, can be directly observed (colour, taste and odour) and can be revealed indirectly by the methods of chemical analysis. It is recognized that hidden biochemical characters are accompanied by morphological divergence for example. Melilotus indica-the correlation of cyanogenic glycoside presence in the white spots on the leaflet.

The inherited metabolism is similar to that of the direct ancestors. The plants are able to adapt themselves to changing conditions and can even change under the influence of sudden or prolonged effect.

Conclusions are that evolution from times and sequences of biosynthesis-and the biochemical process reflects the past.

Ivanov (1915) was the first to recognize the effect of external conditions on the chemical composition of plants.

According to the theory of the 'ecologically directed adaptation mechanism' recorded by Hegnauer (1959), under various ecological and geographical conditions different local plant populations and ecotypes are developed, due to the adaptability of plants.

Ecotypes, according to Hegnauer, are the raw material of evolution. Ecotypes may develop into ecospecies.

The Solanaceae species producing tropane alkaloids, the tropical one's produce Scopolamine, while temperate one accumulate hyoscyamine.

According to the basics of biogenetics this may be regarded as evidence for ecological adaptation during evolution and also for biochemical variability.

Thus, the research work that are being carried out with different collections of medicinal and aromatic plants is of special importance and great significance in the conservation of nature.

The main task now is to preserve the treasure of today's medicinal plants, throughout India and the germ-plasm for posterity.

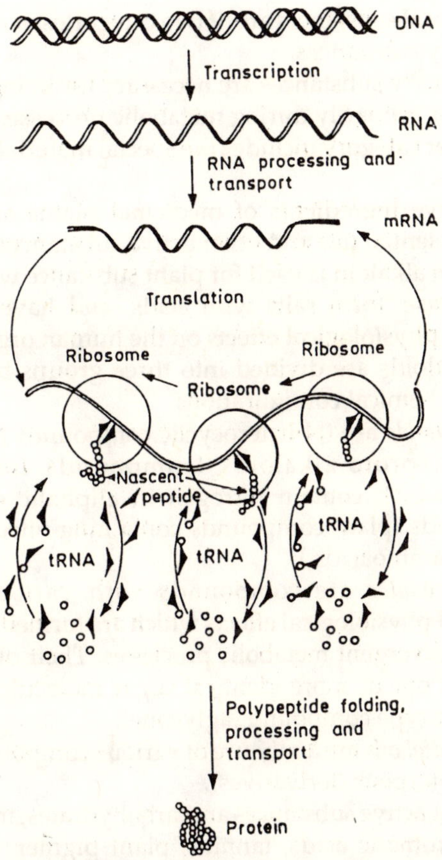

Fig 1 General scheme of protein biosynthesis (DNA→RNA→protein) (Spirin, 1987)

Active Constituents

Medicinal plants contain compounds with special structures and properties (namely, colour, odour, taste, and natural substances).

The natural substances are of two categories namely primary and secondary substances.

The primary substances are necessary for living organisms, and formed of primarily during metabolic processes.

The other category includes the special materials e.g. sterols, fats, alkaloids.

The active ingredients of medicinal plants are alkaloids, glycosides, essential oils and other active substances.

The term alkaloid is used for plant substance which contain nitrogen-as base form salts with acids, and have strong and characteristic physiological effects on the human organism.

The alkaloids are divided into three groups by Hegnauer according to chemical configurations.

True alkaloids are (N-heterocyclic compounds formed from aminoacids), proto-alkaloids (compounds formed from aminoacids, which contain nitrogen in aliphatic chains), and pseudoalkaloids (plant compounds containing nitrogen but not formed from aminoacids.)

The glycosides are compounds with various chemical structures and physiological effects which are formed in a number of extremely divergent metabolic processes. Their only common feature is that one or more identical sugar molecules are bound to a non-sugar type compound (aglycone).

The essential oils are a mixture of various compounds (mainly terpenes, and terpene derivatives).

The plant active substances are carbohydrates, mucilaginous substances, aromatic acids, tannins, plant pigments, Vitamins, bitter substances, sterols, rubber etc.

The Medicinal Plants, Gene Centres

Vavilov named eight primary centres of establishment of cultured plant varieties namely.

(1) India (a) Specific India, (b) India-Malay, (2) China, (3) Central Asia, (4) Near East, (5) Mediterranean, (6) Abyssynian,

(7) South Mexico, Central America (8) South America (a) Peru, Equador, Bolivia (b) Brazil, Paraguay. (9) Europe, (10) North America Medicinal plant families of warmer zone's in the tropics and in the Mediterranean region, e.g. Solanaceae, Rutaceae, Apocynaceae, Labiatae, Rhamnaceae, Fabaceae, Tibaceae, Malvaceae.

The East Asian (Chinese gene centre is rich in medicinal plant species (e.g. Panax pseudoginsengl, Anethum, Sinapis alba originated from the Southern part of the Central Asian Centre.

Ocimum (Tulsi)-is a native of India.

It is remarkable that most of the cultivated medicinal plants originated from the eastern part of the Mediterranean Centre and from the Near East gene Centre, e.g. *Coriander, Pempinella, Foeniculum, Ruta, Salvia officinalis* and one of the ancient cultivated plants, *Calendula officinalis, Hyssopus, Thymus,* and *Digitalis purpurea,* have reached Hungary from the Western parts of the Mediterranean area.

The domestication of tropical plants is closely related to the type of life form and the possibility of changing the life form (e.g. from perennial to annual).

Catharanthus roseus is also a cosmopolitan plant, while the *Solanum laciniatum* is more or less subtropical.

3

Germ-Plasm Studies

Showing *Gene-Complex and presence/absence of active constituents of Indian Species*

	Species	*Gene-Complex*	*Constituents*
1.	*Paeonia emodi* Wall. (Ranunculaceae)	2n = 10	Gly+
2.	*Paeonia officinals* Linn. (Ranunculaceae)	2n = 20	Gly+
3.	*Nigella sativa* Linn (Ranunculaceae)	2n = 12	Gly+
4.	*Cimici-fugia foetida* Linn (Ranunculaceae)	2n = 16	Gly+
5.	*Aconitum napellus* Linn (Ranunculaceae)	2n = 32	Alk++
6.	*Aconitum palmatum* Linn (Ranunculaceae)	2n = 48	Alk+++
7.	*Delphinium ajacis* Linn (Ranunculaceae)	2n = 16	Alk+++
8.	*Delphinum brunonianum* Musk	2n = 16	Alk+
9.	*Helleborus niger* Linn	2n = 32	Alk+++
10.	*Thalictrum folisum* DC (Ranunculaceae)	2n = 14	Alk+
11.	*Thalictrum minus* Linn (Ranunculaceae)	2n = 28	Alk+
12.	*Aquilegia vulgaris* Linn (Ranunculaceae)	2n = 14	Glyco+

	Species	*Gene-Complex*	*Constituents*
13.	*Ranunculus aquatilis* Linn (Ranunculaceae)	2n = 32	Saponins+
14.	*Adonis dahurica* Linn (Ranunculaceae)	2n = 24	glucd+
15.	*Clematis gouriana* Roxb (Ranunculaceae)	2n = 16	Sponins+
16.	*Ceratophyllum demersum* Linn (Ceratophyllaceae)	2n = 24	Alkaloid+
17.	*Nelumbo nucifera* Gaertn (Nymphaecae)	2n = 16	Alkaloid+
18.	*Nymphaea rubra* Roxb. (Nymphaeaceae)	2n = 56	Alkaloid Glycd.
19.	*Nymphaea alba* Linn (Nymphaeaceae)	2n = 112	Glycd
20.	*Nymphaea stellata* Willd (Nymphaeaceae)	2n = 28	Glycd.
21.	*Euryale ferox* Salish (Nymphaeaceae)	2n = 29	Alkaloids+
22.	*Podophyllum emodi* Wall. (Berberidaceae)	2n = 12	Resin+
23.	*Berberis aristata* Dc. (Berberidaceae)	2n = 28	Alkaloid+
24.	*Tinospora cordifolia* Miers (Menispermaceae)	2n = 24	Alkaloid+
25.	*Cocculus laurifoluis* DC. (Menispermaceae)	2n = 26	Alkaloid
27.	*Cocculus villosus* DC. (Menispermaceae)	2n = 38	Alkaloids
28.	*Aristolochia bracteata* Retz (Aristolochiaceae)	2n = 12	Alkaloid+
29.	*Aristolochia indica* Linn. (Aristolochiaceae)	2n = 12	Alkaloids glucoside

	Species	Gene-Complex	Constituents
30.	*Asarum europaeum* Linn (Aristolochiaceae)	2n = 40	Alkaloids+
31.	*Piper longum* Linn (Piperaceae)	2n = 24	ess. Oil
32.	*Piper betle* Linn (Piperaceae)	2n = 32	Glyco
33.	*Piper nigrum* Linn (Piperaceae)	2n = 128	Alk.
34.	*Chloranthus glaber* Makeno (Chloranthaceae)	2n = 30	Alk
35.	*Papaver argemone* Lonn (Papaveraceae)	2n = 42	Alks.++
36.	*Paperver somniferum* Linn (Papaveraceae)	2n = 44	Alkaloids 24+++
37.	*Argemone mexicana* Linn (Papaveraceae)	2n = 28	Alkaloid+
38.	*Meconopsis napalensis* DC (Papaveraceae)	2n = 28	Alkaloid+
39.	*Corydalis sempervirens* R. (Fumariaceae)	2n = 16	Alkaloid+
40.	*Fumaria officinalis* Linn (Fumariaceae)	2n = 28	Alkaloid+
41.	*Capparis sepiaria* Linn (Capparidaceae)	2n = 40	Saponins+
42.	*Capparis spinosa* Linn (Capparidaceae)	2n = 38	glucd.+
43.	*Capparis zeylanica* Linn (Capparidaceae)	2n = 40	Alk.+
44.	*Cleome chelidonii* Linn (Capparidaceae)	2n = 34	Gly.+
45.	*Cleome monophylla* Linn (Capparidaceae)	2n = 22	Gly.+

	Species	*Gene-Complex*	*Constituents*
46.	*Maerua arenaria* Hook f. (Capparidaceae)	2n = 20	Gly.+
47.	*Crataeva religiosa* Linn (Capparidaceae)	2n = 26	Gly.+
48.	*Glynandropsis pentaphylla* (Capparidaceae)	2n = 32	Essential Oil
49.	*Moringa pteryosperma* Gaertn (Moringaceae)	2n = 28	Glyco alkaloids
50.	*Capsella bursa-pastoris* M. (Cruciferae)	2n = 32	Alk.
51.	*Lepidium sativum* Linn (Cruciferae)	2n = 32	Vitc+oil.
52.	*Camellia sinensis* Kuntze (Theaceae)	2n = 40	polyphenols essen oils
53.	*Nasturtium officinale* R.Br. (Cruciferae)	2n = 32	essen oil
54.	*Cheiranthus cheiri* Linn (Cruciferae)	2n = 14	Alk+ Glucd+
55.	*Brassica campestris* Linn (cruciferae)	2n = 20	Oil (glyycendes)
56.	*Brassica juncea* (Linn) Czerns and Coss (Cruciferae)	2n = 36	Esst. Oil
57.	*Brassica napus* Linn (Cruciferae)	2n = 38	Esst Oil
58.	*Raphanus sativus* Linn	2n = 18	esst. oil
59.	*Eruca sativa* Mill (Cruciferae)	2n = 22	Essential oil
60.	*Viola biflora* Linn (Violaceae)	2n = 12	gly. Alk.
61.	*Viola diffusa* Ging (Violaceae)	2n = 26	glycoside

	Species	*Gene-Complex*	*Constituents*
62.	*Sedum multicaule* Wall. (Crassulaceae)	2n = 22	glycoside
63.	*Bryophyllum pinnatum* Pers (Crassulaceae)	2n = 40	Alkaloid
64.	*Dianthus angulatus* Boiss (Caryophyllaceae)	2n = 90	Alkaloid
65.	*Mollugo cerviana* Ser (Ficoidaceae)	2n = 18	glycoside
66.	*Gisekia pharnaceoides* Linn (Ficoidaceae)	2n = 36	Tamnins Glyco
67.	*Trianthema decandra* Linn (Ficoidaceae)	2n = 16	Alk.
68.	*Trianthema pentandria* Linn (Ficoidaceae)	2n = 16	Saponim Alk.
69.	*Portulaca oleracea* Linn (Portulacaceae)	2n = 54	Gly.
70.	*Rumex acetosa* Linn (Polygonaceae)	2n = 12	Oxalates
	(Cultivated)	2n = 12	
71.	*Fagopyrum cymosum* Meissn (Polygonaceae)	2n = 16	Rutin
72.	*Fagopyrum esculentum* Moench (Polygonaceae)	2n = 16	Rutin
73.	*Spinacia oleracea* Linn (Chenopodiaceae)	2n = 12	Oxalic acid.
74.	*Beta vulgaris* Linn (Chenopodiaceae)	2n = 36	iron
75.	*Salicornia brachiata* Roxb (Chenopodiaceae)	2n = 36	Alk.
76.	*Digeria arvensis* Forsk (Amaranthaceae)	2n = 12	Alk.
77.	*Achyranthes bidentata* Blume (Amaranthaceae)	2n = 42	Alk.

	Species	*Gene-Complex*	*Constituents*
78.	*Amarantus blitum* Linn (Amaranthaceae)	2n = 34	KNO_3
79.	*Celosia argentea* Linn (Amaranthaceae)	2n = 72	Betanin
80.	*Celosia cristata* Linn (Amaranthaceae)	2n = 36	Betanin
81.	*Linum usitatissimum* Linn (Linaceae)	2n = 30	Linamarin HCN-glucd
82.	*Balanites aegyptiaca* (Linn) Delile (Zygophyllaceae)	2n = 18	Saponins
83.	*Tribulus terrestris* Linn (Zygophyllaceae)	2n = 48	Alk.
84.	*Oxalis acetosella* Linn (Oxalidaceae)	2n = 28	Oxalic acid
85.	*Impatiens balsamina* Linn (Balsaminaceae)	2n = 14	Glyco
86.	*Lagerstroemia flos-reginae* Linn (Lythraceae)	2n = 44	insulin
87.	*Punica granatum* Linn (Punicaceae)	2n = 18	Alkaloid
88.	*Bougainvillea spectabilis* Linn (Nyctaginaceae)	2n = 34	Gly.
90.	*Mirabilis jalapa* Linn (Nyctaginaceae)	2n = 58	Alk.
91.	*Bixa orellana* Linn (Bixaceae)	2n = 16	Alk.
92.	*Hydnocarpus laurifolia* (Dennst) (Flacourtiaceae)	2n = 22	Hynocarpic acid.
93.	*Tamarix aphylla* Karst (Tamaricaceae)	2n = 24	Tannins
94.	*Passiflora edulis* Sims (Passifloraceae)	2n = 18	HCN

	Species	*Gene-Complex*	*Constituents*
95.	*Momordica balsamina* Linn (Cucurbitaceae)	2n = 22	momordicim
96.	*Melothria heterophylla* Cogn. (Cucurbitaceae)	2n = 48	Glycoside
97.	*Cucurbita maxima* Duch (Cucurbitaceae)	2n = 24	Saponins
98.	*Cucurbita pepo* Linn (Cucurbitaceae)	2n = 40	Phytostearin
99.	*Coccinia indica* W & A. (Cucurbitaceae)	2n = 24	Alk.
100.	*Luffa acutangula* Roxb (Cucurbitaceae)	2n = 26	luffin
101.	*Begonia rex* Putzeys (Begoniaceae)	2n = 34	Glycoside
102.	*Carica papaya* Linn (Caricaceae)	2n = 36	Papain carpaine carposide.
103.	*Opuntia dillenii* Haw (Cactaceae)	2n = 66	Glycosides
104.	*Camellia (Thea) Sinensis* (Theaceae)	2n = 30	Carotene Riboflavin
105.	*Ternstroemia japonica* Thunb (Ternstroemiaceae)	2n = 50	Glycosides
106.	*Dipterocarpus alatus* Roxb (Dipterocarpaceae)	2n = 20	Resin Gystalline acid.
107.	*Hopea odorata* Roxb (Dipterocarpaceae)	2n = 20	Resin
108.	*Eucalyptus globulus* Labill (Myrtaceae)	2n = 22	Oil cineole pinene etc
109.	*Myrtus communis* Linn (Myrtaceae)	2n = 22	Essen oil

	Species	*Gene-Complex*	*Constituents*
110.	*Eugenia jambos* Linn (Myrtaceae)	2n = 54	Glycosides essen oil alk. jambosine
111.	*Psiduim guajava* Linn (Myrtaceae)	2n = 33	eugenol oil
112.	*Osbeckia crinita* Benth (Melastomaceae)	2n = 20	Glyco
113.	*Quisqualis indica* Linn (Combretaceae)	2n = 22	Gum. sterols
114.	*Terminalia catappa* Linn (Combretaceae)	2n = 24	Oil
115.	*Terminalia arjuna* W & A (Combretaceae)	2n = 24	Bark arjunine
116.	*Terminalia belerica* Roxb (Combretaceae)	2n = 24	Tannins
117.	*Terminalia chebula* Retz (Combretaceae)	2n = 24	Tannins
118.	*Hypericum japonicum* Thunp (Hypericaceae)	2n = 16	Tannins
119.	*Calophyllum inophyllum* Linn (Guttiferae)	2n = 32	Oil
120.	*Mesua ferrea* (Guttiferae)	2n = 32	Fls-oil
121.	*Garcina indica* Chois (Guttiferae)	2n = C54	Oil tartaric acid
122.	*Corchorus olitotius* Linn (Tiliaceae)	2n = 14	Vitc Glyco
123.	*Grewia asiatica* Linn (Tiliaceae)	2n = 36	Glyco
124.	*Triumfetta bartramia* Linn (Tiliaceae)	2n = 32	Mucilage

	Species	*Gene-Complex*	*Constituents*
125.	*Theobroma cacao* Linn (Sterculiaceae)	2n = 20	Theobromine Caffeine
126.	*Sterculia foetida* Linn (Sterculiaceae)	2n = 40	Oil
127.	*Pterospermum acerifolium* Willd (Sterculiaceae)	2n = 38	Tannins
128.	*Bombax malabaricum* Schott & End (Bombaceae)	2n = c72	Gum
129.	*Urena lobata* Linn (Malvaceae)	2n = 56	Urease
130.	*Althaea rosea* Cav (Malvaceae)	2n = 56	Oil
131.	*Abutilon crispum* Linn (Malvaceae)	2n = 14	Musulaga
132.	*Sida rhombifolia* Linn (Malvaceae)	2n = 28	Alkaloid
133.	*Hibisccus rosa-sinensis* Linn (Malvaceae)	2n = 144	Gossypetin Glycd. hibsicin
134.	*Gossypuim herbaceum* Linn (Malvaceae)	2n = 26 (= 52)	Glucd etc.
135.	*Euphorbia tirucalli* Linn (Euphorbiaceae)	2n = 20	Euphorbon Ketone latex
136.	*Euphorbia royleana* Boiss (Euphorbiaceae)	2n = 30	latex
138.	*Acalypha hispida* Burm.f. (Euphorbiaceae)	2n = c112	Aclyphine
138.	*Baliospermum axillare* Blume (Euphorbiaceae)	2n = 28	Glyco
139.	*Croton glandulosus* Linn (Euphorbiaceae)	2n = 16	Oil

	Species	*Gene-Complex*	*Constituents*
140.	*Manihot esculenta* Crantz (Euphorbiaceae)	2n = 36	Cyanogentic acid
141.	*Ricinus communis* Linn (Euphorbiaceae)	2n = 20	Oil Ricin Alk : ricinine
142.	*Chrozophora plicata* A. Juss (Euphorbiaceae)	2n = 22	Purgative Oil
143.	*Jatropha curcas* Linn (Euphrobeaceae)	2n = 22	toxic principle curcin fatty oils
144.	*Putranjiva roxburghii* Wall (Euphorbiaceae)	2n = 14	Oil
145.	*Brideldia retusa* Spreng (Euphorbiaceae)	2n = 28	Tannins
146.	*Phyllanthus emblica* Linn (Euphorbiaceae)	2n = 28	Vitc
147.	*Ribes nigrum* Linn (Saxifragraceae)	2n = 32	essen. oil, nophinene, B-naphthol
148.	*Potentilla reptans* Linn (Rosaceae)	2n = 28	tormenol
150.	*Rubus fruticosus* Linn	2n = 14	lactic succinic malic acids Cyanidin monoglucoside
151.	*Geum alatum* Wall (Rosaceae)	2n = 28	essenoil, glucd
152.	*Prunus armeniaca* Linn (Rosaceae)	2n = 16	fatty oil a my gdalin
153.	*Prunus domestica* Linn (Rosaceae)	2n = 48	Oil

	Species	*Gene-Complex*	*Constituents*
154.	*Prunus persica* Batsch (Rosaceae)	2n = 16	Oil
155.	*Cassia auriculata* Linn (Leguminosae)	2n = 16	tannin
156.	*Caesalpenia bonduc* Roxb. (Leguminosae)	2n = 24	bonducin
157.	*Saraca indica* Linn (Leguminosae)	2n = 24	Tannins catechol
158.	*Tamarindus indica*Linn (Leguminosae)	2n = 24	Oxalic acid
159.	*Bauhinia malabarica* Roxb (Leguminosae)	2n = 28	Tannins
160.	*Poinciana pulcherrima* Linn (Leguminosae)	2n = 24	HCN
161.	*Acacea arabica* Linn (Leguminosae)	2n = 52	Tannins
162.	*Albizzia odoratissima* Benth (Black siris) (Leguminosae)	2n = 26	Tannins
163.	*Albizzia procera* Benth (White siris)	2n = 26	Tannins
164.	*Mimosa pudica* Linn (Leguminosae)	2n = 52	Alk. mimosine
165.	*Prosopis spicigera* Linn (Leguminosae)	2n = 28	Alk.
166.	*Lathyrus aphaca* Linn (Leguminosae)	2n = 14	Glyco
167.	*Cicer arcetinum* Linn. (Leguminosae)	2n = 16	Oxalic acetic malicacid Saponins
168.	*Arachis hypogaea* Linn (Leguminosae)	2n = 40	Oil

	Species	Gene-Complex	Constituents
169.	*Desmodium gangeticum* DC (Leguminosae)	2n = 22	Gly
170.	*Lotus corniculatus* Linn (Leguminosae)	2n = 24	Gly
171.	*Medicago sativa* Linn (Leguminosae)	2n = 32.	Gly.
172.	*Trigonella foenum-graecum* Linn (Leguminosae)	2n = 16	Trigonelline
173.	*Melilotus officinalis* Linn (Leguminosae)	2n = 16	Starch
174.	*Melilotus indica* Linn All. (Leguminosae)	2n = 16	Starch Coumarins
175.	*Sesbania aegyptica* Poir (Leguminosae)	2n = 12	Starch
176.	*Indigofera tinctoria* Linn (Leguminosae)	2n = 16	Glycoside
177.	*Glycyrrhiza glabra* Linn (Leguminosae)	2n = 16	Glycoside (Glycyrrhizine)
178.	*Astragalus hamosus* Linn (Leguminosae)	2n = 48	Saponin
179.	*Psoralea corylifolia* Linn (Leguminosae)	2n = 20	Oleoresin
180.	*Tephrosia purpurea* Linn Perse (Leguminosae)	2n = 24	Glucd Rutin
181.	*Baptisia tinctoria* Linn (Leguminosae)	2n = 18	Blue dye
182.	*Rothia trifoliata* Linn (Leguminosae)	2n = 14	Glyco
183.	*Crotalaria juncea* Linn (Leguminosae)	2n = 16	Glyco
184.	*Clitoria ternata* Linn (Leguminosae)	2n = 16	Glyco

	Species	*Gene-Complex*	*Constituents*
185.	*Glycine max* (Leguminosae)	2n = 40	Glyco
186.	*Vigna cylindrica* Skeels (Leguminosae)	2n = 22	Glucd Vicianine
187.	*Arbus precatorius* Linn (Leguminosae)	2n = 22	Abrin glucd
188.	*Mucuna prusiens* Hook (Leguminosae)	2n = 22	Alk. fatty oil
189.	*Cajanus cajan* Linn (Leguminosae)	2n = 44	Starch
190.	*Dolichos lablab* Linn (Leguminosae)	2n = 44	Glycd
191.	*Phaseolus trilobus* Linn (Leguminosae)	2n = 22	Glucd
192.	*Phaseolus vulgaris* Linn (Leguminosae)	2n = 22	Rubidium
193.	*Pueraria tuberosa* DC (Leguminosae)	2n = 24	Glyco
194.	*Erythrina stricta* Roxb (Leguminosae)	2n = 42	Alk.
195.	*Dalbergia sissoo* Roxb (Leguminosae)	2n = 20	Tannins
196.	*Pongamia glabra* Vent (Leguminosae)	2n = 22	Oil
197.	*Derris elliptica* Roxb (Leguminosae)	2n = 24	alk
198.	*Sarcococca pruniformis* Linn (Leguminosae)	2n = 28	Alk
199.	*Populus alba* Linn (Salicaceae) (Salicaceae)	2n = 38	Glucd
200.	*Salix alba.* Linn (Salicaceae)	2n = 76	glucd

	Species	*Gene-Complex*	*Constituents*
201.	*Myrica nagi* Thunb (Myricaceae)	2n = 16	Glyco myricitrin
202.	*Quercus infectoria* Oliv (Fagaceae)	2n = 24	ellagic acid Tannins
203.	*Casuarina equisetifolia* Linn (Casuarinaceae)	2n = 24	Tannins
204.	*Holoptelea integrfolia* Planch (Wlmaceae)	2n = 28	Tannins
205.	*Ficus asperrima* Roxb (Moraceae)	2n = 26	Tannins
206.	*Ficus benghalensis* Linn (Moraceae)	2n = 26	Latex Tannins
207.	*Ficus glomerata* Linn (Moraceae)	2n = 26	Latex
208.	*Ficus indica* Linn (Moraceae)	2n = 26	Latex Tannins
209.	*Ficus carica* Linn (Moraceae)	2n = 26	Proteose Amino-acid
210.	*Artocarpus integra* Linn	2n = 56	Glyco
211.	*Morus alba* Linn (Moraceae)	2n = 42	Glyco Tannins
212.	*Cannabis sativa*Linn (Cannabinanceae)	2n = 40	Cannabinol Cannabinin
213.	*Celastrus paniculatus* Willd (Celastraceae)	2n = 46	Alk Glucd
214.	*Viscum album* Linn (Loranthaceae)	2n = 20	Choline, oleanolic, acid. resin alchohol glucoside.
215.	*Santalum album* Linn (Santalaceae)	2n = 20	Essen Oil Santalon

	Species	Gene-Complex	Constituents
216.	*Balanophora dioica* Linn (Balanophoraceae)	2n = 18	Glyco
217.	*Zizyphus jujuba* Linn (Rhamnaceae)	2n = 40	Glyco
218.	*Zizyphys oenoplia* Mill (Rhamnaceae)	2n = 48	glyco
219.	*Cissus quadrangularis* Linn (Vitaceae)	2n = c45	Cal. oxalate carotene
220.	*Vitis vinifera* Linn (Vitaceae)	2n = 39	gly
221.	*Feronia limonia* Correa (Rutaceae)	2n = 18	Glyco
222.	*Murraya exotica* Linn (Rutaceae)	2n = 18	Glyco
223.	*Citrus medica* Linn (Rutaceae)	2n = 18	Vit.C.
224.	*Citrus limon* Linn (Rutaceae)	2n = 18	Vit. C.
225.	*Citrus aurantifolia* Linn (Rutaceae)	2n = 27	Citric Acid Volatile oil citral limonene
226.	*Aegle marmelos* Corre (Rutaceae)	2n = 36	Marmalosin
227.	*Correa speciosa* (Rutaceae)	2n = 32	Glyco
228.	*Ruta graveolens* Linn (Rutaceae)	2n = 72	Glucd Rutin
229.	*Ailanthus excelsa* Roxb (Simarubaceae)	2n = 62	Glucd Ailantic acid
230.	*Commiphora mukul* Linn (Burseraceae)	2n = 26	Resins

	Species	*Gene-Complex*	*Constituents*
231.	*Melia azedarach* Linn (Meliaceae)	2n = 28	Alkaloids azaridine Tannins resin
232.	*Swietenia mahogoni* Linn (Meliaceae)	2n = 48	Gluco Alka.
233.	*Cedrela tonna* Roxb (Meliaceae)	2n = 56	Bitter sub. red coloury matter ess. Oil
234.	*Cardeospermum halicacabum* Linn (Sapindaceae)	2n = 22	Saponiris
235.	*Litchi chinensis* Linn (Sapindaceae)	2n = 30	Glyco
236.	*Aesculus hippocastanum* Linn (Hippocastanaceae)	2n = 40	Saponins
237.	*Acermono.* Maxim (Aceraceae)	2n = 26	Glyco
238.	*Meliosoma wightii* Linn (Salbiaceae)	2n = 32	Glyco
239.	*Pistacia lentiscus* Linn (Anacardiaceae)	2n = 24	Glyco
240.	*Rhus succedanea* Linn (Anacardiaceae)	2n = 30	Tannins Glyco
241.	*Spondias mangifera* (Anacardiaceae)	2n = 32	Alk.
242.	*Mangifera indica* Linn (Anacardiaceae)	2n = 40	Vit A, C &D.
243.	*Semecarpus anacardium* Linn (Anacardiaceae)	2n = 60	Anacardic Acid
244.	*Anacardium occidentale* Linn (Anacardiaceae)	2n = 42	Cardol. anacardic acid

	Species	*Gene-Complex*	*Constituents*
245.	*Juglan's cinerea* Linn (Juglandaceae)	2n = 32	Oil
246.	*Alangium lamarckii* Linn (Alangiaceae)	2n = 16	Glyco
247.	*Aralia pseudo-gmseng* Benth (Araliaceae)	2n = 48	Saponins
248.	*Carum copticum* Linn (Umbellifereae)	2n = 18	Esst. Oil
249.	*Pimpinella saxifraga* Linn (Umbellifereae)	2n = 18	Esst. Oil
250.	*Apium graveolens* Linn (Umbellifereae)	2n = 22	Esst Oil glucd.
251.	*Hydrocotyle asiatica* Linn (Umbellifereae)	2n = 36	Glyco
252.	*Daucus carota* Linn (Umbellifereae)	2n = 18	Glyco
253.	*Cuminum cyminum* Linn (Umbellifereae)	2n = 14	Esst. Oil
254.	*Coriandrum sastivum* Linn (Umbellifereae)	2n = 22	Oxalic acid ca.
254.	*Ferula assafoetida* Boisss (Umbellifereae)	2n = 22	Gum Resin
255.	*Azalea glabratae* Linn (Rhododendron)	2n = 26	Saponins
256.	*Diospyros lotus* Linn (Ebenaceae)	2n = 30	Tannins Malic acid
257.	*Madhuca latifolia* (Roxb) Macbride (Sapotaceae)	2n = 24	Saponins
258.	*Achras sapota* Linn (Sapotaceae)	2n = 26	Glucd Saponins
259.	*Strychnos nux-vomica* Linn (Loganaceae)	2n = 24	Brucine

	Species	*Gene-Complex*	*Constituents*
260.	*Buddleja asiatica* Lour (Loganiaceae)	2n = 38	Saponins
261.	*Jasminum angustifolium* Vahl (Oleaceae)	2n = 26	Alk.
262.	*Jasminum aruiculatum* Linn (Oleaceae)	2n = 26	alk.
263.	*Jasminum malabaricum* Linn (Oleaceae)	2n = 26	Alk.
264.	*Lochnera rosea* Linn Reichb (A pocynaceae)	2n = 16	Alk
265.	*Allamanda cathartica* Linn (A pocynaceae)	2n = 18	Alk
266.	*Thevetia neriifolia* Juss (Apocynaceae)	2n = 20	Thevetu Gluco
267.	*Plumeria alba* Linn (Apocynaceae)	2n = 36	Alk
268.	*Plumeria rubra* Linn (Apocynaceae)	2n = 36	Glucd Plumeric Acid
269.	*Strophanthus Wallichii* D.C. (Apocynaceae)	2n = 20	Strophan-thin glucd.
270.	*Vallaris heynei* Spreng (Apocynaceae)	2n = 20	Glucd
271.	*Cerbera thevetia* Linn (Apocynaceae)	2n = 20	Glucd
272.	*Carissa carandus* Linn (Apocynaceae)	2n = 22	Alk Sahcylic acid.
273.	*Nerium oleander* Linn (Apocynaceae)	2n = 22	Glucds meriin
274.	*Tabernaemontana coronaria* R.Br (Apocynaceae)	2n = 22	Glucd Alk.

	Species	Gene-Complex	Constituents
275.	*Vinca rosea.* Linn (Apocynaceae)	2n = 46	Alk
276.	*Asclepias curassavica* Linn (Asclepiadaceae)	2n = 22	Glucd
277.	*Ceropegia tuberosa* Roxb. (Asclepidaceae)	2n = 44	Alk.
278.	*Periploca aphylla* Decne (Asclepidaceae)	2n = 22	Resin Alcohol
279.	*Cryptostegia grandiflora* R. Br. (Asclepidaceae)	2n = 24	Latex rubber
280.	*Daemia extensa* R. Br. (Asclepidaceae)	2n = 24	Alk.
281.	*Oldenlandia corymbosa* Linn (Rubiaceae)	2n = 36	Glycu
282.	*Galuim verum* Linn (Leguminosae)	2n = 44	Glucd
283.	*Gardenia campanulata* Roxb (Rubiaceae)	2n = 22	Al.
284.	*Ixora coccinea* Linn (Rubiaceae)	2n = 2	Glyco
285.	*Morinda tinctoria* Linn (Rubiaceae)	2n = 22	Gly morudun
286.	*Randia dumetoruim* Lam (Rubiaceae)	2n = 22	Saponins
287.	*Coffea bengalensis* Linn (Rubiaceae)	2n = 22	Alk. caffeine
288.	*Coffea arabica* Linn (Rubiaceae)	2n = 44	Alkaloide caffeine
289.	*Mussaenda corymbosa* (Rubiaceae)	2n = 22	Glyco
290.	*Pavetta indica* Linn (Rubiaceae)	2n = 22	Glucd

	Species	*Gene-Complex*	*Constituents*
291.	*Rubia cordifolia* Linn (Rubiaceae)	2n = 22	Glucd
292.	*Hamelia patens* Linn (Rubiaceae)	2n = 24	Clucd
293.	*Cinchona ledgereana* Linn (Rubiaceae)	2n = 34	Guinine
294.	*Viburnum foetidum* Wall. (Caprifoliaceae)	2n = 16	Alk.
295.	*Lonicera glauca* Hk. (Caprifoliaceae)	2n = 18	Alk.
296.	*Sambucus ebulus* Linn (Caprifoliaceae)	2n = 36	Cyano-genetic glucd
297.	*Sambucus javanica* Reinw ex. Blume (Caprifoliaceae)	2n = 36	Glucd. oil
298.	*Valeriana officinalis* (Valerianaceae)	2n = 56	oil glucd.
299.	*Launaea glomerata* Hook (Compositae)	2n = 8	Glucd.
300.	*Sonchus oleraceus* Linn (Compositae)	2n = 32	Glucd
301.	*Taraxacum officinale* Weber (Compositae)	2n = 24	Faraxa-sterol phyto-sterols
302.	*Lactuca sativa* Linn (Compositae)	2n = 36	oxalic acid
303.	*Cichorium endivia* (Compositae)	2n = 36	Glucd
304.	*Parthenuim incanum* (Compositae)	2n = 54	Toxic glucd
305.	*Xanthuim strumaruim* Linn (Compositae)	2n = 36	Glucd.

	Species	Gene-Complex	Constituents
306.	*Echpta alba* Hassk (Compositae)	2n = 22	Alk.
307.	*Bidens pilosa* Linn. (Compositae)	2n = 24	Gluc.
308.	*Spilanthes acmella* Murr (Compositae)	2n = 26	Sterols
309.	*Helianthus annuws* Linn (Compositae)	2n = 34	Oil
310.	*Inula graveolens* Desf (Compositae)	2n = 16	
311.	*Carthamus lanatus* Linn (Compositae)	2n = 64	Oil
312.	*Echinops echinatus* Roxb (Compositae)	2n = 32	Oil
313.	*Senecio densiflorus* Wall (Compositae)	2n = 10	Alk
314.	*Notonia grandiflora* Linn (Compositae)	2n = 20	Oil
315.	*Arnica montana* Linn (Compositae)	2n = 38	Oil
316.	*Tagetes erecta* Linn (Compositae)	2n = 24	Oil

4

Germ-Plasm Studies–1967

(Jawaharlal Nehru Ayurvedic Research Institute, Pune)

S.No.	Indian Species	Chromosome Complex
1.	*Annona reticulata* Linn. (Annonaceae) (Ramphal)	2n = 14
2.	*Annona squamosa* Linn (Annonaceae) (Sitaphala)	2n = 14
3.	*Artabotrys odoratissimus* R.Br. (Annonaceae)-(Katchampa)	2n = 16
4.	*Polyalthia longifolia* (Benth & Hookf (Annonaceae) (Devdaru)	2n = 18
5.	*Cinnamomum camphora* Nees & Eberm (Lauraceae) (Karpura)	2n = 24
6.	*Cinnamomum zeylanicum* Blume (Tamalapatra) (Lauraceae)	2n = 24
7.	*Myristica fragrans* Houtt (Myristicaceae) (Jatiphala)	2n = 14
8.	*Taxus baccata* Linn (Taxaceae) (Birmi)	2n = 24
9.	*Cedrus deodara* (Roxb) Loud (Pinaceae) (Devadaru)	2n = 24
10.	*Pinus gerardiana* Wall (Pinaceae) (Rhi, Chida)	2n = 24 2n = 24
11.	*Pinus roxburghu sargent* (Pinaceae) (Chir)	2n = 24

S.No.	*Indian Species*	*Chromosome Complex*
12.	*Cupressus sempervirens* Linn (Saras) (Cupressaceae)	2n = 22
13.	*Juniperus communis* Linn (Aarar) (Cupressacae)	2n = 22
14.	*Ephedra gerardeana* Wall (Asmanid) (Gnetaceae)	2n = 14
15.	*Ephedra intermedia* schrenk & Mey (Oman) (Gnetaceae)	2n = 28
16.	*Michelia champaca* Linn (Champa) Magnoliaceae)	2n = 28
17.	*Annona muricata* Linn (Mullanjaka) (Annonaceae)	2n = 14
18.	*Annona reticulata* Linn (Ramphal) (Annonaceae)	2n = 14
19.	*Annona squamosa* Linn (Sitaphal) (Annonaceae)	2n = 14
20.	*Artabotrys odoratissimus* R.Br. (Harachampaka) (Amonaceae)	2n = 16
21.	*Polyalthia longifolia* Benth & Hookf. (Devadru) (Annonanceae)	2n = 18
22.	*Nigella sativa* (Ranunculaceae)-(Kalijira)	2n = 12
23.	*Cimicifuga foetida* Linn (Jinunti) (Ranunculaceae)	2n = 16
24.	*Caconitum ferox* Wall (Visha) (Ranunculaceae)	2n = 16
25.	*Aconitum chasmanthus* Stapf ex Holmes (Banbalnag) (Ranunculaceae)	2n = 16
26.	*Aconitum heterophyllum* Wall (Ativisha) (Ranunculaceae)	2n = 16
27.	*Aconitum napellus* Linn (Vasha) (Ranunculaceae)	2n = 16

S.No.	Indian Species	Chromosome Complex
28.	*Aconitum palmatum* D. Don (Bikhma) (Ranunculaceae)	2n = 48
29.	*Delphinum ajacis* Linn (Ranunculaceae) (Laskar)	2n = 16
30.	*Delphinum brunonianum* Royle (Laskar) (Ranunculaceae)	2n = 16
31.	*Thalictrum foliolosum* DC (Ratanjota) (Ranunculaceae)	2n = 14
32.	*Anemone obtusiloba* D.Don (Ratanjota) (Ranunculaceae)	2n = 14
33.	*Clematis gouriana* Roxb. (Moriel) (Ranunculaceae)	2n = 16
34.	*Clematis orientialis* Linn (Hushokawal) (Ranunculaceae)	2n = 16
35.	*Clematis smilacifolia* Wall (Vatiyampu) (Ranunculaceae)	2n = 16
36.	*Coptis teeta* Wall (Manira) (Ranunculaceae) (Assam)	2n = 18
37.	*Nolumbo nucifera* Gaertn (Kamala) (Nymphaeaceae)	2n = 16
38.	*Nymphaea stellata* Willd (Krishnakamal) (Nymphaeceae)	2n = 28
39.	*Nymphaea rubra* Roxb. (Raktakambal) (Raktakambal) (Nymphaeceae)	2n = 56
40.	*Herberis aristata* DC (Daruharidra) (Berberidaceae)	2n = 28
41.	*Tinospora cordifolia* Willd Miers (Guduchi) (Menispermaceae)	2n = 24
42.	*Tinospora malabarica* (Lam) Miers (Visha) (Ranunculaceae)	2n = 24
43.	*Cocculus hirsutus* (Linn) Diesl (Vasanvel) (Menispermaceae)	2n = 26

S.No.	Indian Species	Chromosome Complex
44.	*Cocculus pendulus* (Forsk) Diels (Parwatti) (Menispermaceae)	2n = 26
45.	*Aristolochia indica* Linn ((shvari) (ARistolochiaceae)	2n = 12
46.	*Piperbetle* Linn (Tambuli) (Piperaceae)	2n = 32
47.	*Piper nigrum* (Maricha) (Piperaceae)	2n = 128 (Polypoid)
48.	*Piper longum* Linn (Pipali) (Piperaceae)	2n = 24
49.	*Piper chaba* Hunter (Chavika) (Piperaceae)	2n = 24
50.	*Papaver argemone* Linn (Poppy) (Papaveraceae)	2n = 42
51.	*Paperver sonmiferum* Linn (Ahiphenum) (Papaveraceae)	2n = 22
52.	*Argemone mexicana* Linn (Srigala-Kantaka) 9Papaveraceae)	2n = 28
53.	*Corydalis govaniana* Wall (Bhutakesi) (Fumariaceae)	2n = 12
54.	*Fumaria indica* Pugsley (Pit. papara) (Fumariaceae)	2n = 28
55.	*Fumaria officinalis* Linn (Pit. Papara) (Fumariaceae)	2n = 32
56.	*Capparis sepiaria* Linn (Kakadani) (Capparidaceae)	2n = 40
57.	*Cleome chelidonni* Linn.f (Ubhitalvani) (Capparidaceae)	
58.	*Crataeva religeosa* Linn (Capparidaceae)	2n = 26
58.	*Gynandropsis gynandra* (Linn) Briquet (Surjavarta) (Capparidaceae)	2n = 32

S.No.	Indian Species	Chromosome Complex
60.	*Moringa oleifera* Lam (Sobhajana) (Moringaceae)	2n = 28
61.	*Capsella bursa-pastoris* Medic (Cruciferae)	2n = 16
62.	*Lepidium sativum* Linn (Chandrashura (Cruciferae)	2n = 32
63.	*Nasturtium officinale* R.Br. (Cruciferae) (Piriya halim)	2n = 16
64.	*Brassica campestris* Linn (Cruciferae) (Kalisarson)	2n = 20
65.	*Brassica juncea* (L) Czern & Coss (Asia-rai) (Cruciferae)	2n = 36
66.	*Brassica nigra* (Linn) kech (Raisarisha (Cruciferae)	2n = 36
67.	*Raphanus sativus* Linn (Crufierae) (Mulaka)	2n = 18
68.	*Viola biflora* Linn (Violaceae)	2n = 12
69.	*Viola odorata* Linn (Banafshah) (Violaceae)	2n = 40
70.	*Kalanchoe pinnata* Pers. (Crassulaceae) (Zakhmhaiyat)	2n = 34
71.	*Bergenia ligulata* (Wall) Engl. (Patharchur-Pashanabheda)	2n = 34
72.	*Drosera burmanni* vahl. (Droseraceae) (Mukhajali)	2n = 20
73.	*Drosera peltata* Sm. (Droseraceae) (Mukhajali)	2n = 40
74.	*Saponaria vaccaria* Linn (Caryophyllaceae) Musna	2n = 28
75.	*Dianthus anatolicus* Boiss (Caryo phyllaceae) (Kanturiyan)	2n = 90

S.No.	Indian Species	Chromosome Complex
76.	*Mollugo cerviana* Ser. (Ghimsag) (Ficoidaceae)	2n = 18
77.	*Mollugo nudicaulis* Lam. (Pappadagam) (Ficoidaceae)	2n = 54
78.	*Mollugo oppositifolia* Linn (Phanija) (Ficoidaceae)	2n = 36
79.	*Gisekia pharnaceoides* Linn (Valuka) (Ficoidaceae)	2n = 36
80.	*Trianthema decandra* Linn (Punarnavi) (Ficoidaceae)	2n = 16
81.	*Portulaca oleracea* Linn (Portulacaceae) (Lonika)	2n = 54
82.	*Portulaca guadrifida* Linn (Portulacaceae) (Upadyki)	2n = 48
83.	*Poligonum aviculare* Linn (Polygonaceae) (Nisomali)	2n = 40
84.	*Polygonum viscosum* Linn (Polygonaceae)	2n = 22
85.	*Polygonum flaccidum* Meissn (Polyonaceae)	2n = 44
86.	*Rheum emodi* Wall (Polygonaceae) (Revatchini)	2n = 22
87.	*Rheum officinale* Baillon (Polygonaceae)	2n = 44
88.	*Phytolacca acinosa* Roxb. (Phytolaccaceae) (Matazor)	2n = 36
89.	*Spinacia oleracea* Linn (Palak) (Chenopodiaceae)	2n = 12
90.	*Beta vulgaris* Linn (Palanki) (Chenopodeaceae)	2n = 18
91.	*Chenopodium album* Linn (Vastak) (Chenopodiaceae)	2n = 36

S.No.	*Indian Species*	*Chromosome Complex*
92.	*Digera muricata* (L) Mart. (Luta mahawaria) (Amaranthaceae)	2n = 16
93.	*Achyranthes aspera* Linn (Latjira) (Amaranthaceae)	2n = 32
94.	*Achyranthes bidentata* Blume (Apamarga) (Amarathaceae)	2n = 42
95.	*Celosia argentea* Linn (Safoid murgha) (Amaranthaceae)	2n = 72
96.	*Celosia cristata* Linn (Mayurashikha) (Amaranthaceae)	2n = 36
97.	*Basella alba* Linn (Putika) (Basellacea)	2n = 48
98.	*Linum usitatissimum* Linn (Alasi, Alsi) (Linaceae)	2n = 30
99.	*Balanites aegyptiaca* (Linn) Delile (Ingudi) (Simarubaceae)	2n = 18
100.	*Tribulus terrestris* Linn (Gokshura) (Zygophyllaceae)	2n = 24
101.	*Averhoa carambola* Linn (Karmal) (Oxalidaceae)	2n = 24
102.	*Oxalis acetosella* Linn (Amlika) (Oxalidaceae)	2n = 22
103.	*Averrhoa carambola* Linn (Karmal) (Oxalidaceae)	2n = 24
104.	*Impatiens balsamina* Linn (Gulmendi, Dupati) (Balsaminaceae)	2n = 14
105.	*Lagerstroemia flos-reginae* Retz. (Phurush, Dhayti) (Lythraceae)	2n = 44
106.	*Punica granatum* Linn (Dadima) (Punicaceae)	2n = 18
107.	*Bouganivillea spectabilis* Linn (Boganivilla) (Nyctaginaceae)	2n = 34

S.No	Indian Species	Chromosome Complex
108.	*Mirabilis jalapa* Linn (Krishnapeli) (Gulabbas) (Nyctaginaceae)	2n = 58
109.	*Dillenia indica* Linn (Bhavya, Chalta) (Dilleniaceae)	2n = 32
110.	*Bixa orellanga* Linn (Sindure, Latkan) (Bexaceae)	2n = 16
111.	*Flacourtia indica* Merr. (Bilangra, Kaher) (Flocourteaceae)	2n = 22
112.	*Hydnocrpus laurifolia* (Dennst) (Kowte, Kava) (Flacourtiaceae)	2n = 48
113.	*Hydnocarpus anthelmintica* Parre (Chaulmoogra) (Flacourtiaceae)	2n = 24
114.	*Tamarix aphylla* Karst (Laljhav, Raktajhav) (Tamaricaceae)	2n = 24
115.	*Passiflora foetida* Linn (Mukkopeera) (Passifloraceae)	2n = 20
116.	*Cucumis melo* Linn (Kharbuja) (Cucurbitaceae)	2n = 24
117.	*Momordica balsamina* Linn (Mokha, Kurelo-jangro) (Cucurbitacea)	2n = 22
118.	*Momordica charantia* Linn (Sushavi, Karela) (Cucurbitaceae)	2n = 22
119.	*Trichosanthes anguina* Linn (Chichenda, Pandolu) (Cucurbitaceae)	2n = 22
120.	*Melothria heterophylla* Cogn. (Kudari, Gometta) (Cucurbetaceae)	2n = 48
121.	*Coccinia indica* W & A (Bimba) (Cucurbitaceae)	2n = 24
122.	*Carica papaya* Linn (Papaya) (Papai) (Caricaceae)	2n = 36
123.	*Opuntia dillenu* Haw (Vidara, Nagphana) (Cactaceae)	2n = 66

S.No.	*Indian Species*	*Chromosome Complex*
124.	*Camellia assamica* (Linn)-Kuntze (Gernsteromiaceae-Thaceae) (Tea-Cha)	2n = 30
125.	*Eucalyptus globulus* Labill (Nigiri, Karpura maram) (Myrtaceae)	2n = 22
126.	*Eugenia jambolana* Lam. (Syn. Syzygium cuminilin) (Myrtaceae) (Jambu, Jamin)	2n = 22
127.	*Terminalia catappa* Linn (Jangli badam) (Combretaceae)	2n = 24
128.	*Garcinia indica* Chois (Kokum) (Guttiferae)	2n = 54
129.	*Corchorus acutangulus* Linn (Kalasaka) (Tiliaceae)	2n = 14
130.	*Corchorus olitorius* Linn (Koshta, Tankia) (Tileaceae)	2n = 14
131.	*Bombax cieba* Linn (Sali) (Bompacaceae)	2n = 72c
132.	*Althacea officinalis* Linn (Gulkhairo) (Malvaceae)	2n = 42
133.	*Sida rhombifolia* Linn (Atibala) (Malvaceae)	2n = 28
134.	*Sida acuta* Burm (Bala) (Malvaceae)	2n = 28
135.	*Sida spinosa* Linn Nagabala (Malvaceae)	2n = 28
136.	*Hibiscus abelmoschus* Linn (Latakasturika, Mushdana) (Malvaceae)	2n = 72
137.	*Hibiscus rosa-sinensis*Linn (Jasvand) (Malvaceae)	2n = 144
138.	*Euphorbia hirta* Linn (Dudhi) (Euphorbiaceae)	2n = 28
139.	*Croton tiglium* Linn (Jayapala, Jamalgota) (Euphorbiaceae)	2n = 20

S.No.	Indian Species	Chromosome Complex
140.	*Ricinus communis* (Eranda) (Euphorbeaceae)	2n = 20
141.	*Chrozophora plicata* A Juss (Syn.: Chrozophora protrata Dalz (Shadevi) (Euphorbaceae)	2n = 22
142.	*Jatropha curcas* Linn (Mogalierenda) (Euphorbeaceae)	2n = 22
143.	*Jatropha gossypifolia* Linn (Kariturukaharlu) (Euphorbeaceae)	2n = 22
144.	*Jatropha multifeda* Linn (Vishabhadra) (Euphorbeaceae)	2n = 22
145.	*Putranjiva roxburghu* Wall (Putranjiva) (Euphorbeaceae)	2n = 14
146.	*Bridelia retusa* Spreng (Khaja, Geio)	2n = 28
147.	*Phyllanthus emblica* Linn Syn: Emblica officinalis Gaertn (Ovla) (Euphorbeacea)	2n = 28
148.	*Ribes nigrum* Linn (Nabar) (Saxifragaceae)	2n = 16
149.	*Potentilla fruticosa* Linn (Spanjha) (Rosaceae)	2n = 14
150.	*Prunus amygdalus* Batasch (Badam) (Rosaceae)	2n = 16
151.	*Cassia auriculata* Linn (Tarwar Tarwad (Leguminosae)	2n = 16
152.	*Cassia fistula* Linn (Suvarnaka, Amaltas) (Leguminosae)	2n = 24
153.	*Cassia tora* Linn (Takla, Tagarai) (Leguminosae)	2n = 26
154.	*Cassia angustifolia* Vahl (Sonamukhi) (Leguminosae)	2n = 28

S.No	Indian Species	Chromosome Complex
155.	*Caesalpinia bonducella* Fleming (Kuberakshi, Karanja Sagarghota)	2n = 24
156.	*Saraca indica* Linn (Ashoka)	2n = 24
157.	*Tamarindus indica* Imli (Leguminosae)	2n = 24
158.	*Bauhinia purpurea* Linn Vanaraja (Rhatakanchan) (Leguminosae)	2n = 28
159.	*Bauhinia variegata* Linn (Kachnar) (Leguminosae)	2n = 28
160.	*Acacia catechu* Willd. (Khair) (Leguminosae)	2n = 26
161.	*Acacia arabica* Willd Babal (Leguminosae)	2n = 52
162.	*Albizzia odoratissima* Kala siris (Leguminosae)	2n = 26
163.	*Mimosa pudica* Linn (Lajja, Lajwanti) (Leguminosae)	2n = 52
164.	*Prosopis spicigera* Linn (Shami) (leguminosae)	2n = 26
165.	*Lathyrus sativus* Linn (Sandika) (Leguminosae)	2n = 14
166.	*Arachis hypogaea* Linn (Mungphali) (Leguminosae)	2n = 40
167.	*Desmoduin gangeticum* DC (Shalaparni) (Leguminosae)	2n = 22
168.	*Lotus hirsutus* Linn (Leguminosae) (Padma)	2n = 24
169.	*Trigonella foenum-graecum* Linn (Leguminosae) (Methi)	2n = 16
170.	*Trigonella corniculata* Linn (Malya) (Leguminosae)	2n = 16

S.No.	Indian Species	Chromosome Complex
171.	*Melilotus indcia* (Linn) Ali (Banamethika) (Leguminosae)	2n = 16
172.	*Sesbania aegyptiaca* Poir (Jayanti) (Leguminosae)	2n = 12
173.	*Indigofera tinctoria* Linn (Yashti-madhu) (Leguminosae)	2n = 16
174.	*Glycyrrhiza glabra* Linn (Yashti-madhu) (Leguminosae)	2n = 16
175.	*Psoralea corylefolia* Linn (Babuchi) (Leguminosae)	2n = 20
176.	*Tephrosia purpurea* (Linn) Pers. (Sharapunkha) (Leguminosae)	2n = 24
177.	*Crotalaria verrucosa* Linn (Shanapushpi) (Leguminosae)	2n = 16
178.	*Crotalaria juncea* Linn (Sana) (Leguminosae)	2n = 16
179.	*Clitoria ternatea* Linn (Aparajita) (Leguminosae)	2n = 16
180.	*Glycine max* Merr. (Bhat) (Leguminosae)	2n = 40
181.	*Vigna cylindrica skeel* (Rajamasha (Leguminosae)	2n = 22
182.	*Abrus precatoruis* Linn (Gunja) (Leguminosae)	2n = 22
183.	*Mucuna prurita* Hook (Atmagupta) (Leguminosae)	2n = 22
184.	*Cajanus indicus* Linn (Adhaki) (Leguminosae)	2n = 22
185.	*Dolichos biflorus* Linn (Kulatha) (Leguminosae)	2n = 24
186.	*Erythrena varegata* Linn (Pangara, Mandar) (Leguminosae)	2n = 42

S.No.	*Indian Species*	*Chromosome Complex*
187.	*Dalbergia latifolia* Roxb. (Shishapa, Sitsal) (Leguminosae)	2n = 20
188.	*Pongamia pinnata* (Linn) Merr. (Karanjal) (Leguminosae)	2n = 22
189.	*Pterocarpus marsupuim* Roxb. (Bibla, Bijasar) (Leguminosae)	2n = 44
190.	*Salix alba* Linn (Bis) (Salicaceae)	2n = 76
191.	*Betula alnoides* Buch-Ham. (Bhujpatra) (Betulaceae)	2n = 28
192.	*Casuarina equisetifolia* Linn (Janglisaru) (Casuarinaceae)	2n = 24
193.	*Ficus bengalensis* Linn (Vata Vad.) (Moracae)	2n = 26
194.	*Ficus carica* Linn (Anjira) (Moraceae)	2n = 26
195.	*Ficus glomerata* Linn (Udumbara) (Moraceae)	2n = 26
196.	*Ficus religiosa* Linn (Pipal) (Moraceae)	2n = 26
197.	*Ficus tscela* Roxb (Pimpri) (Moraceae)	2n = 26
198.	*Artocarpus heterophyllus* Lam. (Panasa) (Moraceae)	2n = 56
199.	*Morus alba* Linn (Tut.) (Moraceae)	2n = 28
200.	*Morus indica* Linn (Tut) (Moraceae)	2n = 28
201.	*Morus rubra* Linn (Tuti) (Moraceae)	2n = 28
202.	*Urtica dioica* Linn (Bichu) (Urticaceae)	2n = 48

S.No.	Indian Species	Chromosome Complex
203.	*Cannabis sativa* Linn (Cannabinacae) Bhang Charas Ganja	2n = 20
	Ganja	2n = 40
204.	*Celastrus paniculatus* Willd (Celastraceae) (Kanguni, Malkangni)	2n = 46
205.	*Santalum album* (Chandan) (Santalaceae)	2n = 20
206.	*Zizyphus officinale* Rosc. (Adrak) (Zingiberaceae)	2n = 24
207.	*Cissus quadrangularis* Linn (Asthisanhara) (Vitaceae)	2n = 45
208.	*Vitis vinefera* Linn (Draksha) (Vitaceae)	2n = 38
209.	*Feronia elephantum* Correa (Kavitha) Kavit (Rutacaea)	2n = 18
210.	*Murraya paniculata* (L) Jack (Kamini, Marchula) (Rutaceae)	2n = 18
211.	*Aegle marmelos* Corr. (Bilva, Bael) (Rutaceae)	2n = 36
212.	*Ruta graveolens* Linn (Rutaceae) (Somalata Sadab)	2n = 72
213.	*Zanthoxylum acanthopodium* DC (Turmra) (Rutaceae)	2n = 70
214.	*Ailanthus excelsa* Roxb. (Maharukha, Maharimba) (Simarubaceae)	2n = 62
215.	*Comiphora mukul* Engl. (Burseraceae)	2n = 26
216.	*Melia azedarach* Linn (Maha-nimba) (Meliaceae)	2n = 28
217.	*Melia azadirchta* Linn (Meleaceae) (Nim)	2n = 28

S.No.	*Indian Species*	*Chromosome Complex*
218.	*Cedrela toona* Roxb (Meliaceae) (Nandivreksha) (Tun)	2n = 56
219.	*Cardiospermum halicacabum* Linn (Karnasphota) (Sapindaceae)	2n = 22
220.	*Aesculus hippocastanum* Linn (Pu) (Hippocastanaceae)	2n = 40
221.	*Rhus chinensis* Mill (Tatri) (Anacardeaceae)	2n = 30
222.	*Spondias magnifera* Willd (Anacardiaceae) (Amrataka)	2n = 32
223.	*Mangifera indica* Linn (Ami) (Anacardeaceae)	2n = 40
224.	*Semecarpus anacardium* Linn.f (Bhallika) (Biba) (Anacardeaceae)	2n = 60
225.	*Anacardium occidentale* Linn (Kaju) (anacardeaceae)	2n = 42
226.	*Juglans riga* Linn (askhrot) (Juglandaceae)	2n = 32
227.	*Alkanguim lamarckii* Thwaites (Syn. A. Salvifolium Wang (Alangeaceae)	2n = 16
228.	*Carcum copticum* Benth & Hook.f. (Syn. Trachyspermum animi (Linn) Spraque (Umbelleferae) Kala Zira.	2n = 18
229.	*Carum Carvi* (Shea jira) (Umbelliferae)	2n = 20
230.	*Pimpinella anisum* Linn (Shetapusapa, Saonf) Umbelleferae)	2n = 20
231.	*Anethum graveolens* Kurz Dill (Umbelliferae) (Satapuspi)	2n = 32
232.	*Apium graveolens* Linn (Ajamoda) (Umbelliferae)	2n = 22

S.No.	*Indian Species*	*Chromosome Complex*
233.	*Hydrocotyl asiatica* Linn (Centella asiatica (L) Urban (Umbelliferae, Brahm.	2n = 18
234.	*Daucus carota* Linn (Gajar) (Umbrelliferae)	2n = 18
235.	*Cuminum cyminum* Linn. (Jira, Zira) (Umbelliferae)	2n = 14
236.	*Coriandrum sativum* Linn (Dhane) (Umbelliferae)	2n = 22
237.	*Rhododendron anthopogon* D.Don (Ericaceae) (Tazak-tsum)	2n = 26
238.	*Madhuca indica* J.G.Emel. (Sy. M. latifolia (Roxb.) Mcbride (*yn. Bassica lalifolia* Roxb. (Mahua) (Sapotaceae)	2n = 24
239.	*Achras zapota* Linn (Sapotaceae) (Chiku)	2n = 26
240.	*Strychnos nux-vomica* (Kuchla, Visha-mushti) (Loganeaceae)	2n = 24
241.	*Jasminum arborescens* Roxb. (Chamli) (Oleaceae)	2n = 26
242.	*Thevetia peruviana* (Pers.) (Syn.: T. nerifolia Juss (Pila-kaner (Apocynaceae)	2n = 18
243.	*Plumera alba* Linn (Kananakaravira) (Apocynaceae)	2n = 36
244.	*Plumeria rubra* Linn (Devaganagalu), (Goburchampa) (Apocynaceae)	2n = 36
245.	*Strophanthus wallichi* A.DC (Karvi (Apocynaceae)	2n = 40
246.	*Carissa carandas* Linn (Karaunda) (Apocynaceae)	2n = 22

S.No	Indian Species	Chromosome Complex
248.	*Tabernaemontana coronaria* (Tagar) (Apocynaceae)	2n = 22
249.	*Vinca rosea* Linn (Sadaphuli) (Apocynaceae)	2n = 32
250.	*Asclepeas curassavica* Linn (Kurki) (Asclepeadaceae)	2n = 22
251.	*Ceropegia bulbosa* Roxb. (Khapparkadu Galot) (Asclepidaceae)	2n = 44
252.	*Periploca aphylla Decne* Berri (Asclepeadaceae)	2n = 22
253.	*Cryptostegia grandi flora (Roxb)* R. Br. (Vilayti-vakhandi)_ (Asclepeadaceae)	2n = 24
254.	*Daemia extensa* R. Br. Syn. Pergularea extensa R.Br (Chagulbanti, Utarni) (Asclepeadaceae)	2n = 24
255.	*Oldenlandia corymbosa* Linn (parpata, pati (Rubeacead)	2n = 36
256.	*Gardenia gummifera* Linn.f. (Dikamali) (Rubeaceae)	2n = 22
257.	*Ixora coccinea* Linn (Bandhuka) (Rubeaceae)	2n = 22
258.	*Morinda tinctoria* Roxb. (Ach, Achchuka) (Rubeaceae)	2n = 22
259.	*Randia dumetorum* Lam. (Mandana, Mainphal) (Rubeaceae)	2n = 22
260.	*Cephaelis ipecacuanha* A. Rich (Rubeaceae)	2n =44
261.	*Coffea arabica* Linn (Coffe) (Kafi) (Rubeaceae)	2n = 44
262.	*Rubia cordifolia* Linn (Majistha) (Rubiaceae)	2n = 22

S.No.	*Indian Species*	*Chromosome Complex*
263.	*Cinchona ledgeriana* Moens (Quinine) (Rubeaceae)	2n = 34
264.	*Viburnum foetdum* Wall (Shirporna, Jaya) Narvel, Lequminosae	2n = 16
265.	*Lonicera glauca* H.K.f. (Sheva) (Carprifoleaceae)	2n = 18
266.	*Sambucus ebulus* Linn (Mushkeara) (Caprifoleaceae)	2n = 36
267.	*Valeriana hardwickii* Wall (Taggar) (Valerianaceae)	2n = 28
268.	*Valeriana officinalis* Linn (Kalavala) (Valereanaceae)	2n = 56
269.	*Lactuca sateva* Linn (Compositae)	2n = 16
270.	*Cichorium intybus* Chicory (Compositae) (Kasni)	2n = 18
271.	*Eclipta alba* Hask (Compositae) (Bhringaraja, Maka	2n = 22
272.	*Spilanthes acmela* Murr (Akarkara (Compositae)	2n = 26
273.	*Meleanthus annus* Linn (Suryaphul) (Compositae)	2n = 34
274.	*Inula indica* Linn (Rasan) (Compositae)	2n = 20
275.	*Chrysanthemum parthenium* Linn (Guldaude, Akurkura, Sevanti) (Compositae)	2n = 18
276.	*Chrysanthemum parthenium* Linn (Compositae)	2n = 18
277.	*Elephantopus scaber* Linn (Gojihva, gobhi) (Compositae)	2n = 22

S.No.	*Indian Species*	*Chromosome Complex*
278.	*Ageratum conyzoides* Linn (Uchunti, Osari) (Compositae)	2n = 40
279.	*Swertia chirata* Buch-Ham (Chereta) (Genteanaceae)	2n = 24
280.	*Plumbago indica* Linn Chitraka (Plumbagenaceae)	2n = 14
281.	*Plantago ovata* Linn (Isabgol) (Plantageneace)	2n = 8
282.	*Carthamus lanathus* Linn (Compositae)	2n = 64
283.	*Echinops echinatus* Roxb. (Utakanta, Utanti) (Compositae)	2n = 16
284.	*Senecio echinatus* Linn (Chitawala) (Compositae)	2n = 60
285.	*Tridax procumbens* Linn (Chitawala) (Compositae)	2n = 60
286.	*Arnica montaria* Linn (Compositae) (Himalayas)	2n = 38
287.	*Tagetes erecta* Linn (Gendu) (Compositae)	2n = 24
288.	*Artemisia absinthium* Linn (Vilayati afsantin) (Compositae)	2n = 18
289.	*Artemisia absinthium* Linn (Akarakara) (compositae)	2n = 18
290.	*Pedalium murex* Linn (Baragokhru) (Pedaleaceae)	2n = 16
291.	*Sesamum indicum* Linn (Tila (Pedaleaceae)	2n = 26
292.	*Martynia annua* Linn (Bichu (Pedaleaceae)	2n = 36
293.	*Hygrophita spinosa* T. Andero Syn. Asteracanthax longifolia Nees (Acanthaceae)	2n = 12

S.No.	*Indian Species*	*Chromosome Complex*
294.	*Adhatoda vaseca* Nees Adulasa (Acanthaceae)	2n = 34
295.	*Vitex agnus castus* Linn (Panjangusht) (Verbenaceae)	2n = 24
296.	*Vitex negundo* Linn (Nergundi (Verbenaceae)	2n = 24
297.	*Lippia nodiflora* Mich (Vashira) (Verbenaceae)	2n = 36
298.	*Lantana camara* Linn (Ghaneri (Verbenaceae)	2n = 44
299.	*Heliotropium indicum* Linn Hastisunde (Boragenaceae)	2n = 24
300.	*Cestrum nocturnum* Linn (Jasmine) (Solanaceae)	2n = 16
301.	*Nicoteana tabacum* Linn (Tambaku)	2n = 24
302.	*Withania somnifera* Dunal Ashvakanda (solanaceae)	2n = 48
303.	*Cuscuta reflexa* Roxb. A marvel (Convolvulaceae)	2n = 28
304.	*Convolvulus arvensis* Linn Hiranpade (Convolvulaceae)	2n = 50
305.	*Cesiacoromandeleana* Vahl Bhutakeshi (Scrophuraceae)	2n = 34
306.	*Clerodendron indicum* (Linn) Ktze Bharange (Verbenaceae)	2n = 48
307.	*Rosmarinus officinalis* Linn Rusmari (Labeatae)	2n = 24
308.	*Coleus forskohlii* Linn Karpurvale (Labeatae)	2n = 28
309.	*Thymus serpyllum* Linn Masho (Labeatae)	2n = 24

S.No.	*Indian Species*	*Chromosome Complex*
310.	*Mentha arvensis* Linn Pudena (Labeatae)	2n = 74
312.	*Lavandula bipinata* O.Ktze Sarpnocharo (Labeatae)	2n = 24
313.	*Salvia officinalis* Linn (Laliatae) (Labeate)	2n = 14
314.	*Salvia dumetorum* Linn Labeeatae)	2n = 14
315.	*Salvia officinalis* Linn Salbea (Labeatae)	2n = 14
316.	*Ocimum basilicum* Linn Munjareki (Labeatae)	2n = 48
317.	*Ocimum gratissimum* Linn Ramtulsi (Labeatae)	2n = 64
318.	*Ocimum sanctum* Linn Tulsi (Labeatae)	2n = 64
319.	*Costus speciosus* Sm. Kemka (Zingiberaceae)	2n = 36
320.	*Zingiber officinale* Rose Adrak (Zingoberaceae)	2n = 22
321.	*Eletteria cardamomum* Maton Ela (Zingeberaceae)	2n = 48
322.	*Hedychium specatum* Ham ex smith Karchura (Zingeberaceae)	2n = 34
323.	*Urginea indica* Kunth Vana-palandam (Labaceae)	2n = 20

References

1. Darlmgton C.D. and K. Mather, (1950), Gene, Plants and People, Allen and Wnwin.

2. La Cour L.F., (1947), The Handling of Chromosomes, Allen and Hnwin.
3. Darlungton C.D., (1932), Chromosomes and Plant Breeding, Macmillan.
4. Hornok. L., (1992), Cultivations and Processing of Medicural Plants, John Wiley and Sons, New York.
5. Karnick C.R., (1994), Pharmacopoeial Standards of Herbal Plants, Vol. I and II.

5

New Herbal Drugs in Offings

1. *Glycyrrhizin* (Yashtimadhu)

It is well-known that quite a large number of people suffer from chronic diseases without appropriate therapies One of such disease is liver disorders.

There are a number of natural drugs that have curative effects on liver disorders in traditional medicine.

Recent progress in the study of traditional drugs has resulted in the isolation of a number of active principles including anti-hepatotoxic constituents. Clinical effects were evaluated for liver protective activity on a scientific basis, using double-blind tests (cf. Handa, S.S., Sharma, A., Chakraborti, K.K. (1986), Fitoterapia 57, 307).

Glycyrrhizin is used to sweeten decoctions to mitigate the action of drastic drugs and to relieve pain caused by muscle contraction.

Glycyrrhizin is one of the main components of licorice root. It consists of one molecule of glycyrrhetinic acid and two molecules of glucuronic acid.

Because glycyrrhizin contains glucuronic acid. Earlier it assumed that glycyrrhizin has an antidotal action. Based on this view point-a preparation of glycyrrhizin has been used for allergies and detoxification in the field of dermatology in Japan since 1948.

During the course of such clinical use, glycyrrhizin preparation were found to be effective for chronic hepatitis and lever currhosis.

Examination of the effect of glycyrrhizin and Gal N-induced liver damage demonstrated that glycyrrhizin inhibited liver cell injury but did not reverse reduced protein synthesis.

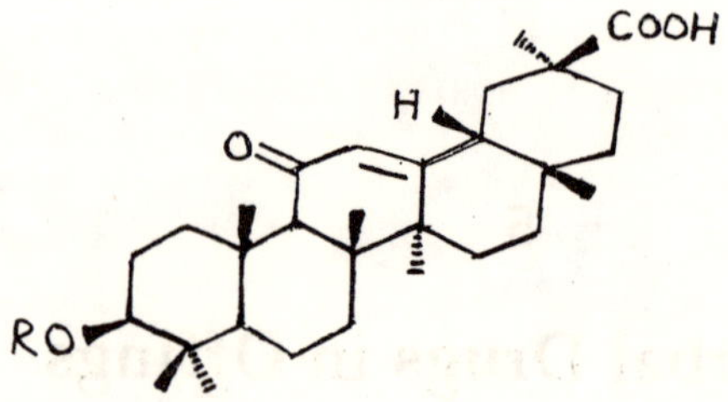

Glycyrrhizin = R = D - Glc A - B
(1 → 2) D-Glc A

Glycyrrhctinic acid R = H

Uridine improved morphological lesions and also reduced protein synthesis (Okita et al 1975-Okitak, Noda.K. Kondo.N and Mizuta, M. (1975)-Kanzo **16** : 620).

Further, on Gal N-Induced liver damage glycyrrhizin has been confirmed to have inhibitory action against CCl_4-, benzene hexachloride, mitomycin c and polychlorinated biphenyl-induced liver lensions by means of histological observations (Watari 1977-Minophagen Med. Rev 22, 170).

It has now been found that using primary cultured rat hepatocytes it was found that glycyrrhizin showed protective action against hepatocytotoxity induced by CCl_4 (cf. Kiso. et al 1983-Plant Medica **49** : 222).

Investigations of the structure activity relationships in glycyrrhizin and its analogues in CCI_4-and Gal N-induced cell damage indicated, that among the analogues, glycyrrhetinic acid and glycyrrhizin exhibited their most prominent effects on cytotoxicity induced by each haptotoxin (cf Kiso et al 1984 Planta Medica **50** : 298).

There is evidence that CCI_4 is first metabolized by drug-metabolizing enzymes (represented by Cytochrome P-450 in the liver endoplasmic reticulum) to the highly reactive CCl_3 radical, which induces lipid peroxidation, covalent binding to macromolecules and inhibition of the calcium pump of microsomes leading to lever damage (Recknagel 1983 : Life Sa **33**:401).

The mechanism of inhibitory activity of glycyrrhizin and glycyrrhetinic acid against CCl_4-induced liver lesions was investigated, demonstrating that the anti-hepatotoxic action of glycyrrhizin and glycyrrhetinic acid is not dependent on its steroidal action because the artificial 18-glycyrrhetinic acid, which has an oxygen function on the E-mg, thus adopting a similar conformation to that of prednisolone, revealed significantly stronger anti-inflammatory activity than that of the natural 18-glycyrrhetinic acid, which exhibited much less anti-hepatotoxic action.

Further, from the results obtained by determining the effects of these substances on the initial steps in the sequence of events leading to CCl_4-induced liver lesions, it was seen that the antioxidative actions of glycyrrhizin and glycyrrhetinic acid participate in the ante hepatotoxic activity. (Kiso et al 1984).

Immunological mechanisms play an important role in the induction and progression of human liver disease.

A model of experimental chronic active hepatitis in rabbits has been produced by immunization with human liver specific lipo-protein (LSP) which is a plasma-membrane associated antigen complex (Meyer Zum Buschenfelde and Muscher 1972. Br. J. Exp. Pathol. **55** : 498) and anti-LSP antibody was detected in the sera of immunized animals (Hopf. et al, 1974) and also in the sera of patients with various liver diseases, (Hopf. et al 1976 N. Engl. J. Med. **294** : 578).

Further studies have shown that the level of anti-SLP, antibody correlated with the magnitude of liver injury. (Jensen et al 1978) indicating that anti-LSP anti-body may be involved in the pathogenesis of liver disease. These observations suggest that patients with chronic active hepatitis are in a slate hypersensitive to LSP.

Anti-body-dependent cell-mediated cyto-toxicity (ADCC) has been recorded to take part in liver cell damage in hepatitis. Indeed, using isolated rabbit hepatocytes are target cells, has been demonstrated that lymphocyte cytotoxicity for hepatocytes is observed in non-T cell populations from patients with chronic active hepatitis and is blocked by the addition of LSP (Cochrane et al 1976). It is also observed that liver cell damage may be induced by activated macrophages infiltrating into the liver tissue of patients, because various lymphokines, including macrophage activating factor are produced by peripheral blood lymphocytes (PBL) from patients with liver diseases, especially chronic active hepatitis, when stimulated with LSP (Mizoguchi et al 1981. Hepato-gastro-enterology **28** 250). The effect of glycyrrhizin on immunological induced lever damage, an investigated in vitro studies using isolated rat live cells.

Thus, an ADCC reaction was induced by co-culture with isolated liver cells coated with anti-LSP antibody and peripheral blood mononuclear cells as effector cells. When the culture supernatant separated from the ADCC reaction mixture and was added to freshly prepared liver cells, protein synthesis in liver cells was reduced.

Pretreatment of liver cells with glycyrrhizin prevented the reduction of protein synthesis significantly, but not in a dose-dependent manner (Mizoguxhi et al 1985 Abstr. Pap. 21st Annu Meet Jpn. Soc. Hepatal.)

Similarly, activated macrophage-mediated cytotoxicity was produced by addition of cultured super-natant of peritoneal exudate macrophages, activated by lipopolysaccharide, to freshly prepared isolated liver cells.

Reduced protein synthesis was observed in the supernatant-treated culture.

When the liver cells were pretreated with limited doses. The most effective concentration of glycyrrhizin in ADCC and activated macro-phage mediated cytotoxicity was 20 µg/ml, and excess amounts of glycyrrhizin were not beneficial.

It is concluded from above results that glycyrrhizin may protect liver cells from immunologically induced liver injuries (Mizoguchi et al 1985).

The enhancement of antibody production by glycyrrhizin has also be investigated by in vitro methods.

When mono-nuclear cells from human peripheral blood was stimulated with pokeweed mitogen (PWM) in the presence of glycyrrhizin, polyclonal antibody production was significantly enhanced as compared with the case in which mononuclear cells were stimulated with PWM alone. Because the culture supernatant from glycyrrhizin-treated monocytes also caused an enhancement of antibody production was attributed, at least partially, to the activation of monocytes.

By gel filtration, the active component contained in the

culture supernatant of glycyrrhizin-treated monocytes was assumed to be interleukin I because the fractionated substance was similar in molecular size to inter leukin I and caused an increase in DNA synthesis of phytohemagglutinin (PHA0 - stimulated thymocytes.

The findings suggest that glycyrrhizin may have an enhancing effect on antibody formation through the production of inter leukin I. (cf. Mizoguchi et al 1984).

The glycyrrhizin preparation (SNMC) presently employed for clinical trials. It consists of glycyrrhizin (40 mg). Cysteine (20 mg), and glycine (400 mg) in 20 ml of physiological saline.

Investigation of the effect of glycyrrhizin on virus growth showed that Glycyrrhizin inhibited the growth of several DWA and RNA viruses but had no effect on protein synthesis and replication of uninfected cells.

According to Pompei et al 1979 (Nature-London 281, 689) glycyrrhizin inactivated herpis simplex virus particles.

Clinical trials of antihepatotoric and therapeutic effects of glycyrrhizin in liver diseases-it shows lowering effect of serum transaminase levels.

II Vasicine

Adhatoda vasic Nees (Acanthaceae)

The extract of *A. vasica* is an official preparation included in large number of cough remedies.

Vasicine was said to be active bronchodilator. Latter it was found it is found to be uterine stimulant activity and which is lost when vasicine is metabolized by the liver.

Ayurvedic literature, revealed that midwives used *A. vasica* leaves to control post-partum hemorrhage.

Arya V.P. (1981) (cf. Drugs of the future **6** 373) listed vasicine as an oxytocic and abortiafacient drug.

Clinical evaluation of vasicine was published in 1981. (Arya 1981)-showing in vivo effects of this compound in human beings.

9 to 10 post-maturity or incoordination uterine contraction cases were reported to have delivered normally when vasicine

20 mg in 500 ml of dextrose) used found to induce labour (Atal 1980-Chemistry and Pharmacology of Vasicine-a new Oxytocic and Abortifacent, 155 pp. RR Lab Jammu-Tawi)

Post-partum bleeding was checked in 60 cases in which vasicine (50-10 mg diluted with saline, was administered. Wakhloo et al 1980 (India J. Pharmaol **12** : 129) carried out clinical, toxicological studies in 24 patients-postmortem hospital inpatient received 0.5 to 16 mg doses of vasicine in 500 ml of saline infused over, 3 hrs. 16 mg to 12 volunteers clearly effective intra-amninotically administered abortifacient dose.

(III) Anti-Viral

Phyllanthus niruri Linn (Sans: Bhumyamalaki, Jar-amla)
Phyllanthus reticulatus Poir (Sans: Krishna kambhoji / Panjoli)
Phyllanthus simplex Retz (Bhwavali)
Phyllanthus urinaria Linn. (Sans : Tam ravatti, Lalmunda janvali) are *Antiviral* use

It is useful against jaundice, liver diseases, skin eruptions, viral diseases (mumps, small pox, chicken pox, herpes dengue and influenza.

Relief to pruritis

It is also used against edema or dropsy., kidney, bladder stones. It is also useful in malaria, intermittent fevers.

$$LP_{50} > 1g/kg$$

(cf David. Wander et al. (1995) : Usage and bioassays in *Phyllanthus* (Euphorbiaceae) IV Clustering of Antiviral use and other effects : *Jour of Ethnopharmacology* 45 : 1-18.

IV Anti-Entamoeba histolytica

Youvraj R. Sohni et al (1995).

The antiamoebic effect of a crude drug formulation of herbal extracts against *Entamoeba histolytica* in vitro and in vivo.

Journal of Ethnopharmacology 45 : 43-52

The anti-amoebic effect of a crude drug formulation against Entamoeba histolytica was studied.

It comprises of five medicinal herb namely *Boerhavia diffusa, Berberis aristata Tinospora cordifolia, Terminalia chebula* and *Zmgiber officinale*

The ethanotic extracts were found to whit - in varying degrees-some of the enzymes of axenic *E. Histolytica.*

V. Anti-Salmonella typhi (Anti Typhoid herbal drug)

Youvraj R. Sohni et al. (1995) : Ptophylactic therapy of *Salmonella typhi* septicemia in mice with a traditionally prescribed crude drug formulation

Journal of Ethnopharmacology 45 : 141-147.

Drug consisted of

Boerhaavia diffusa-roots
Tinospora cordifolia-stem
Berberis aristata-roots
Terminalia chebula (fruits)
Zingibir officinale (rhizome)
Azadirchta indica (bark)
Trichosanthes dioica (Vine)
and *Picrorrhiza kurraoa* (roots)

It was observed that Picrorrhiza kurrooa and others etc. inhibited the growth of the test organism *salmonella typhi* septicemia in mice. A prophylactic dose regimen induced a significantly protective effect.

Phyllanthus is extensively used to treat jaundice and inhibits hepadnavirus DNAp, effects on chronic infection with hepatitis Bveries (HBV) or related viruses.

VI. S. Manonmani et al (1994)

Biochemical evaluation of the antiulcerogenic effect of Cauvery 100 (an ayurvedic formulation) in rats *Journal* of

Ethnopharmacology 42 : 1-5 Cauvery-100. Composition of the drug was :

1. *Emplica officinalis* L. (Euphorbiaceae) fruit-50mg.
2. *Cuminum cyminum* L. (Umbelliferae)-fruit-50mg.
3. *Trema orientalis* (L.) Blume-Wrtecaceae root-50mg.
4. *Vitis vinfera* L. (Vitaceae) fruit-50mg
5. *Carum carvi* L. (Umbelliferae) for-100mg
6. *Withania somnifera* (L) Dunal (Solanaceae) Root-100
7. *Eclipta alba* (L.) Hassk. Compositae (herb)-50 mg
8. *Embelia tibes* Burm. f. (Myrisinaceae) fr.-100mg
9. *Citrug limon* (L) Burm. f. (Rutaceae) fr rund-50mg
10. Picrorrhiza kurrooa Benth, Scrophulaseaceae Rt-100mg
11. Glycyrrhiza glapra L. (Papilionaceae) stem-100mg
12. Aegle marmelos (L) Corr. (Rutaceae) root-50.
13. Zingiber officinale Rose (Zingiberaceae) rhiz-50mg

This regulates both the acid out put and mucous secretion and highly antiulcerogenic

VII. Skin disease-Pityriasis versicolor-Cassia alata

S. Damodaran et al (1994) : A study on the therapeutic efficacy of *Cassia alata* Linn. Leaf extract against Pityriasis

Jour. of Ethnopharmacology 42 : 19-23

The leaf extract of *Cassia alata* was found clinically effective anti fungal and it treated Pityriasis versicolor, with out side-effects

VIII. Nyclanthes arbor-tristis L.

Anju Puri et al. (1994) Immunostimulant activity of *Nyctanthes* arbortristis Linn Jour. Ethnopharmacology 42: 31-37

Nyctanthes arbortristis L. (Oleaceae) widely used in traditional medicinal systems of India-has been reported to possess hepatoprotective, antileishmanial, antiviral and anti fungal activities.

In the present study strong stimulation of antigen specific and non-specific immunity, as evidenced by increases in humoral and delayed type hypersensitivity (DTH) response to sheep red blood cells (SRBC) and in the macrophage migration index (MMI) has been demonstrated in mice fed with 50% ethanolic extract of seeds, flowers and leaves of this plant.

Maximum activity was found in the seeds in which the active principle appear to be associated with *lepids.*

In flowers and leaves, major activity was found in the aqueous fraction of 50% Ethanol extract.

The immunostimulant substances found in N. arbor-tristis L. are likely to playa role in its anti amoebic, antileishmanial, antiviral and certain other activities.

IX. Rauvalfa Canescens

Madawala, P.G. et al (1944):

Studies on the sedative activity of crude extract of root bark of Ranvolfia canescens on rats.

Jour. of Ethnopharmacology 42 : 63-65

Ranvolfia serpentina Benth (Apocyanaceae) roots have been used as hypnotics and Sedatives in neuropsychiatric disorders in anxiety states and in epilepsy.

The possible sedative activity of Rauvolfia canescens root extract was evaluated using the rat hole board technique.

Crude extract of R. Canescens has sedative properties None showed signs of toxicity at the effective dose (50mg/kg).

Several indole alkaloids-namely ajmaline, yohimbme, isoreserpine, corynanthine, deserpidine-a new alkaloid have been isolated from root book. The sedative property is due to reserpone type of alkaloids present.

Root extracts of *E. canescens* also possesses sedative activities like *R. serpentme* Roots.

X. Hyperlipidaemea

Nelumbo nucifera

Bergitee la Cour et al (1995)

Traditional Chinese medicine in treatment of hyperlipidaemia.

Jour. of *Ethnopharmacology* 46 : 125-129

Nelumbo nucifera has a cholesterol and phospholipid reducing effect Gunostemma pentaphylla (Thunb) Mark has strengthening and lipid reducing effect. (Chinese Academy of Medical Sciences et al. 1990).

XI. Daucus carota L.

Anupam Bishayee et al (1995)

Hepatoprotective activity of Carrot (Daucus carota L.) against Carbon tetrachloride intoxication in mouse lever :
Journal of Ethnopharmacology 47: 69-74

The present investigation demonstrates that the various biochemical changes produced in the serum and liver of mouse by CCl_4 treatment were reversed, prevented by pretreatment with carrot extract.

Carrot juice is rich in carotenes Carotenes include B-carotene, carotene, V-carotene, lycopene, cryptoxanthin, leutein abscisic acid trsporic acid., B-apo-carotenals, crocetin, polar cartoenoids e.g. Violaxanthin

These compounds have the potential to minimise the deleterious effects of free radicals including the perory radicals and hence ranked as hepato protective agents.

Curcuma longa

R. Selvam. et al. (1995):

The anti-oxidant activity of Tumeric (Curcuma longa)
Journal of Ethnopharmacoloty 47 : 59-67.

The turmeric anti-oxidant protein (TAP) has been isolated from aqueous extract of turmeric.

Current interest has been focused on the potential role of anti-oxidants and anti-oxidant enzymes in the treatment and prevention of certain diseases.

Curcuma longa-possess anticancer, anti-coagulative and anti-hepatotoric principles.

It dissolves urinary calculus, controls diabetes

Calotropis procera* R. Br. and *Semecarpus anacardum L.F.

Smit H.F. et al. (1995)

Ayurvedic herbal drugs with possible cytostatic activity

Jour. of Ethnopharmacology 47 : 75-84

Extracts of the flowers of calotropis procera (Art) R.Br. (Asclepiadaceae) and the nuts of Semecarpus anacarduim Lf. (Anacardiaceae) display a strong cytotoric effect with IC_5 values of 1.4 mg/ml & 1.6 mg/ml respectively.

Celastrus paniculatus (Malhangni) Nalini K. et al (1995) : Effects of Celastrus paniculatus on passive avoidance performance and bogenic amini turnover in albim rats.

Jour. of Ethnopharmacology 47 : 101-108

Celastrius paniculatus Willd. the oil extracted from seeds is said to have effect on the CNS and has beneficial effects in psychiatric patients Celastrus oil therapy is used in mentally retarded children produced improvement in I.Q. Celastrus oil causes an overall decrease in the turnover of all the three central monoamines and implicate the involvement of these ammergic systems in the learning and memory process.

Ashwagandha, Ginseng

Anuradha Grandhi (1994) : A comparative pharmacological investigation of Ashwagandha and Ginseng.

Journal of Etho-pharmacology 44 : 131-135

Ashwagandha and Ginseng were tested for pharmacological

activities namely anti-stress activity and swimming endurance test in mice.

Ginseng showed 3.2378% steroids while Ashwagandha-2.8245% steroids in roots Another mechanism is antiserotoginic activity of Ashwagandha leading to stimulation of appetite and enhancing food intake. Ashwagandha is found beneficial in old age of variety of geriatric problems. *Ginseng* abuse syndrome-adverse effect. No side effects reported in case of Ashwagandha.

Eugenia uniflora Linn

Schapoval et al. (1994) Evaluation of some pharmacological activities of Eugenia uniflora Linn

Journal of Ethnopharmacology 44 : 137-142.

It is anti-inflammatory, increases pen to barbaritol sleeping time.

Useful in treating gout, urinary tract infections.

Pippali

Agarwal A.K. et al. (1994).

Management of giardeasis by an immumo-modulatory herbal drug

Pippali rasayan

Journal of Ethnopharmacology 44 : 143-146.

Giardiasis is a common gastro-intestinal infection caused by a protozoal parasite—*Giardia lamblia.*

In present study the immuno-modulatory and anti-giardial activities of pippali rasayana-an Ayurvedic herbal medicine was prepared from Piper longum L. (Piperaceae) and Butea monosperma (lam) Kuntze (Leguminosae. It was tested on mice and found that chronic dysentery and worm infestation-disappeared and 98% recovery from the Infection.

Curcuma longa and Catechin

Prevention of Cancer. Azuine M.A. et al (1994) Adjuvant chemopreention of experimental Cancer : Catechin and dietary turmeric in forestomach and oral cancer models.

Jour of Ethnopharmacology 44 : 211-217.

Catechin in drinking water and dietary turmeric inhibited the tumor burden and tumor incidence in Swiss mice. These findings suggest that catechin and turmeric which are regularly consumed natural products are effective in golden hamsters as chemopreventive agents.

Kroes, B.H. et al (1993)

Termentation in traditional medicine : the impact of Wood fordia fruticosa flowers on the immunomodulatory activity and alcohol and sugar contents of Nimba-arishta.

Jour of Ethnopharmacology 40 : 117-125

The use of Woodfordia flowers in model preparations resulted in a substantial increase of the inhibition of both human complement activity and chemi-luminescence generated by zymosanstimualted human polymorphonuclear leukocytes.

It was established that the increased biological activity was not due to microbial interference, but to immuno-active constituents released from the Woodfordia flowers.

Andrographis paniculata

Visen, P.K.S., et al (1993):

Andro-grapholide protects rat hepatocytes against paracetamol-induced damage

Jour of Ethnopharmacology 40 : 131-136.

The active constituents isolated from Andrographis paniculata, showed protective activity against paracetamol-induced toxicity. Silymarin is standard hepato-protective agent.